Created by <u>BabyDreamers.net</u>

♥   Designed In New Zealand

Free Book Offer:

Get How to be a Super Mom For Free

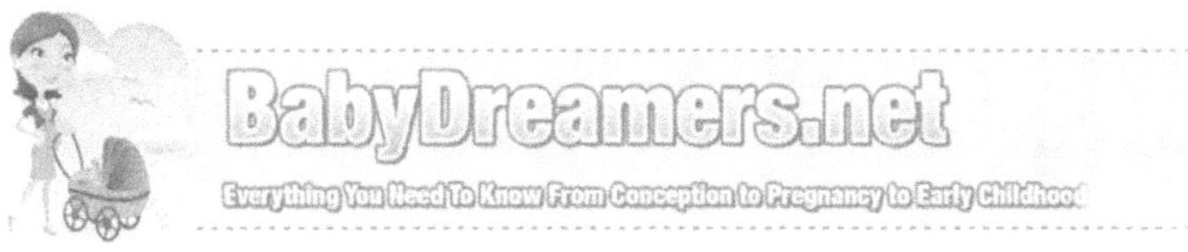

A Short Read is a type of book that is designed to be read in one quick sitting.

These no fluff books are perfect for people who want an overview about a subject in a short period of time.

Table of Contents

The Role of Male Fertility in Conception

The role of male fertility in the process of conception is of utmost importance and has a significant impact on the successful outcome of pregnancy. Male fertility refers to the ability of a man to impregnate a woman and father a child. It involves various factors such as sperm production, sperm health, hormonal balance, sexual health, lifestyle factors, age, medical conditions, and environmental factors.

Sperm production plays a crucial role in male fertility. The testes are responsible for producing and storing sperm cells. The process of sperm production, known as spermatogenesis, involves the continuous production of millions of sperm cells every day. These sperm cells are necessary for fertilization to occur and initiate the conception process.

In addition to sperm production, sperm health is also vital for successful conception. Healthy sperm refers to sperm cells that have optimal characteristics and are capable of fertilizing an egg. Factors such as sperm count, sperm motility, and sperm morphology contribute to sperm health. Sperm count refers to the number of sperm cells present in a semen sample. Higher sperm count increases the chances of conception. Sperm motility refers to the ability of sperm cells to move and swim towards the egg for fertilization. Good sperm motility is crucial for successful fertilization. Sperm morphology refers to the shape and structure of sperm cells. Abnormalities in sperm morphology can hinder the chances of conception.

Furthermore, hormonal balance plays a significant role in male fertility. Hormones such as testosterone, follicle-stimulating hormone (FSH), and luteinizing hormone (LH) are essential for the proper functioning of the reproductive system. Testosterone levels influence sperm production and overall reproductive health. FSH stimulates the production of sperm cells, while LH plays a role in the release of testosterone. Imbalances in these hormones can affect male fertility and the ability to conceive.

Sexual health is another crucial aspect of male fertility in the process of conception. Conditions such as erectile dysfunction can affect the ability to achieve and maintain an erection, making it difficult to engage in sexual intercourse and potentially hindering conception. Additionally, sexually transmitted infections (STIs) can have detrimental effects on male fertility and increase the risk of infertility.

Lifestyle factors also play a significant role in male fertility and conception. Habits such as smoking and excessive alcohol consumption can impair sperm production and quality, reducing the chances of successful fertilization. A healthy diet and proper nutrition are essential for optimal sperm health and overall reproductive function. Regular exercise and maintaining a healthy weight also contribute to male fertility.

Age is another factor that impacts male fertility. As men age, their fertility declines, and the chances of conception decrease. Advancing paternal age is associated with an increased risk of genetic abnormalities and potential complications during pregnancy.

Certain medical conditions can also affect male fertility and the ability to conceive. Conditions such as varicocele, a swelling of the veins in the scrotum, can interfere with sperm production and quality. Genetic disorders and hormonal disorders can also have a significant impact on male fertility.

Environmental factors can also influence male fertility and conception. Exposure to chemicals and radiation can affect sperm production and quality, potentially reducing the chances of successful fertilization.

In conclusion, male fertility plays a crucial role in the process of conception and has a significant impact on the success of pregnancy. Understanding the various factors that contribute to male fertility and taking steps to maintain optimal reproductive health can increase the chances of successful conception and a healthy pregnancy.

Sperm Production

Sperm production, also known as spermatogenesis, is a crucial process in male fertility. It is the process by which the male body creates mature sperm cells that are capable of fertilizing an egg during conception. Understanding the intricacies of sperm production is essential in comprehending its role in male fertility.

The process of sperm production begins in the testes, specifically in the seminiferous tubules. These tubules contain specialized cells called spermatogonia, which are the precursor cells for sperm. Through a series of divisions and differentiations, spermatogonia develop into spermatocytes, which then undergo meiosis to produce haploid spermatids. These spermatids further mature and transform into fully functional sperm cells.

During sperm production, several factors influence the quality and quantity of sperm produced. These include hormonal regulation, genetic factors, and environmental influences. Hormones such as follicle-stimulating hormone (FSH) and luteinizing hormone (LH) play a crucial role in stimulating and regulating the process of sperm production. Genetic factors can affect the overall health and viability of sperm, while environmental factors such as exposure to chemicals or radiation can have detrimental effects on sperm production.

Overall, sperm production is a complex process that plays a vital role in male fertility. Understanding the intricacies of this process can help individuals and couples better comprehend the factors that contribute to successful conception and take necessary steps to optimize male fertility.

Sperm Health

Sperm health plays a crucial role in the process of conception and is essential for successful pregnancy. The factors that contribute to healthy sperm are multifaceted and can greatly impact the chances of conception.

One of the key factors in sperm health is sperm count. Sperm count refers to the number of sperm present in a given sample. A higher sperm count increases the likelihood of successful fertilization. Low sperm count, also known as oligospermia, can significantly decrease the chances of conception. It is important for men to maintain a healthy lifestyle and avoid factors that can negatively impact sperm count, such as smoking, excessive alcohol consumption, and exposure to certain environmental toxins.

Sperm motility is another crucial aspect of sperm health. Motility refers to the ability of sperm to move effectively and swim towards the egg for fertilization. Poor sperm motility, also known as asthenospermia, can hinder the chances of conception. Factors that can influence sperm motility include hormonal imbalances, certain medications, and underlying health conditions. It is important for men to maintain a balanced hormonal profile and seek medical advice if they suspect any issues with sperm motility.

Sperm morphology, or the shape and structure of sperm, is also important for healthy sperm and successful conception. Abnormal sperm morphology, known as teratospermia, can impact the ability of sperm to penetrate and fertilize the egg. Factors such as genetic abnormalities, hormonal imbalances, and exposure to environmental toxins can contribute to abnormal sperm morphology. Maintaining a healthy lifestyle and seeking medical advice for any underlying conditions can help improve sperm morphology and increase the chances of conception.

In conclusion, the factors that contribute to healthy sperm are crucial for successful conception. Sperm count, motility, and morphology all play significant roles in the fertilization process. It is important for men to prioritize their overall health and make lifestyle choices that support optimal sperm health. By understanding and addressing these factors, couples can increase their chances of conceiving and starting a family.

Sperm Count

The sperm count is a crucial factor in determining male fertility and plays a significant role in the chances of conception. Sperm count refers to the number of sperm cells present in a semen sample. It is measured through a semen analysis, which examines various parameters of sperm health.

A healthy sperm count is typically considered to be around 15 million sperm cells per milliliter of semen. However, it's important to note that the ideal sperm count may vary depending on the specific fertility guidelines of different healthcare professionals. A low sperm count, also known as oligospermia, can significantly reduce the chances of successful conception.

There are several factors that can impact sperm count. These include lifestyle choices, such as smoking, excessive alcohol consumption, and poor diet. Additionally, certain medical conditions, such as hormonal disorders or testicular infections, can also affect sperm production and lead to a low sperm count.

It's important for individuals who are trying to conceive to be aware of their sperm count and take steps to optimize it. This may involve making lifestyle changes, such as quitting smoking, reducing alcohol intake, and adopting a healthy diet. In some cases, medical interventions may be necessary to address any underlying conditions that may be affecting sperm count.

Overall, understanding the importance of sperm count in determining male fertility and conception is crucial for individuals who are hoping to start a family. By taking proactive steps to optimize sperm count, individuals can increase their chances of successful conception and parenthood.

Sperm Motility

Sperm motility plays a crucial role in the process of fertilization and ultimately, successful pregnancy. Motility refers to the ability of sperm to move and swim effectively, allowing them to reach and penetrate the egg for fertilization to occur. Without proper motility, the chances of conception are significantly reduced.

There are several factors that can affect sperm motility. One key factor is the shape and structure of the sperm cells. Sperm with abnormal morphology may have difficulty swimming properly, hindering their ability to reach the egg. Additionally, the health of the sperm cells is important for optimal motility. Sperm that are damaged or have poor quality may struggle to swim effectively.

Other factors that can impact sperm motility include hormonal imbalances, certain medical conditions, and lifestyle choices. Hormonal imbalances, such as low testosterone levels, can affect the overall health and motility of sperm. Medical conditions like varicocele, a condition characterized by enlarged veins in the scrotum, can also impair sperm motility.

Lifestyle choices, such as smoking, excessive alcohol consumption, and poor diet, can have a negative impact on sperm motility. These factors can contribute to oxidative stress and inflammation, which can damage sperm cells and reduce their ability to swim effectively. On the other hand, maintaining a healthy lifestyle with regular exercise and a balanced diet can support optimal sperm motility.

In conclusion, sperm motility is a critical factor in successful fertilization and pregnancy. Understanding the role of sperm motility and addressing any issues that may affect it can significantly improve the chances of conception. By maintaining a healthy lifestyle, addressing hormonal imbalances, and seeking appropriate medical care, couples can increase their chances of achieving a successful pregnancy.

Sperm Morphology

Sperm morphology refers to the size, shape, and structure of sperm cells. While it may seem like a small detail, it plays a crucial role in male fertility and the chances of successful conception. The shape of sperm cells is important because it affects their ability to swim and fertilize an egg.

Abnormal sperm morphology, also known as teratozoospermia, can significantly impact male fertility. When a large percentage of sperm have abnormal shapes, it can make it difficult for them to reach and penetrate the egg. This can decrease the chances of fertilization and hinder the process of conception.

There are various factors that can contribute to abnormal sperm morphology. These include genetic abnormalities, exposure to toxins or radiation, hormonal imbalances, and certain medical conditions. Additionally, lifestyle factors such as smoking, excessive alcohol consumption, poor diet, and obesity can also affect sperm morphology.

To determine sperm morphology, a semen analysis is typically conducted. During this test, the shape and structure of sperm cells are examined under a microscope. The World Health Organization (WHO) has established criteria for normal sperm morphology, with a minimum percentage of normally shaped sperm required for optimal fertility.

If a man has abnormal sperm morphology, it does not necessarily mean that he is infertile. However, it may decrease the chances of conception and increase the time it takes to achieve pregnancy. In some cases, assisted reproductive techniques such as in vitro fertilization (IVF) may be recommended to overcome fertility challenges related to sperm morphology.

In conclusion, sperm morphology plays a significant role in male fertility and the process of conception. Understanding and addressing any abnormalities in sperm shape is essential for couples trying to conceive. By maintaining a healthy lifestyle, seeking medical advice when necessary, and exploring fertility treatments, couples can increase their chances of successful pregnancy.

Hormonal Balance

Hormonal balance plays a crucial role in male fertility and has a significant impact on the ability to conceive. Hormones are chemical messengers in the body that regulate various bodily functions, including reproductive health. When it comes to male fertility, certain hormones play a key role in the production and maturation of sperm, as well as the overall reproductive process.

One of the primary hormones involved in male fertility is testosterone. Testosterone is responsible for the development and maintenance of male reproductive tissues, including the testes and prostate gland. It also plays a vital role in sperm production and maturation. Low testosterone levels can negatively affect sperm quality and quantity, reducing the chances of successful conception.

Another hormone that plays a crucial role in male fertility is follicle-stimulating hormone (FSH). FSH is produced by the pituitary gland and stimulates the production of sperm in the testes. It helps regulate the maturation of sperm cells and ensures their proper development. Imbalances in FSH levels can impact sperm production and quality, affecting male fertility.

Luteinizing hormone (LH) is another hormone that influences male fertility. LH is responsible for stimulating the production of testosterone in the testes, which is essential for sperm production. It also triggers the release of mature sperm into the reproductive tract. Imbalances in LH levels can disrupt the hormonal balance, leading to fertility issues.

It is important to maintain a healthy hormonal balance for optimal male fertility. Hormonal imbalances can be caused by various factors, including certain medical conditions, lifestyle choices, and age. Consulting with a healthcare professional and undergoing hormone level testing can help identify any imbalances and guide appropriate treatment options.

In conclusion, hormonal balance plays a significant role in male fertility and has a direct effect on the ability to conceive. Testosterone, follicle-stimulating hormone (FSH), and luteinizing hormone (LH) are key hormones involved in sperm production and maturation. Maintaining a healthy hormonal balance is essential for optimal male fertility and increasing the chances of successful conception.

Testosterone Levels

Testosterone levels play a crucial role in male fertility and the ability to conceive. Testosterone is the primary male sex hormone, responsible for the development and maintenance of male reproductive tissues and secondary sexual characteristics. It is produced in the testes and plays a vital role in the production of healthy sperm.

Optimal testosterone levels are essential for spermatogenesis, the process of sperm production. Low testosterone levels can lead to a decrease in sperm count, motility, and morphology, all of which are important factors in male fertility. It is important for men to maintain balanced testosterone levels to maximize their chances of successful conception.

Several factors can influence testosterone levels, including age, lifestyle, and underlying medical conditions. As men age, testosterone levels naturally decline, which can impact fertility. Additionally, certain lifestyle factors, such as smoking, excessive alcohol consumption, poor diet, and lack of exercise, can negatively affect testosterone production.

Medical conditions, such as hormonal disorders and genetic disorders, can also disrupt testosterone levels and impair male fertility. It is crucial for men to address any underlying medical conditions and maintain a healthy lifestyle to optimize testosterone levels and improve their chances of conception.

In conclusion, understanding the significance of testosterone levels in male fertility is essential for couples trying to conceive. Maintaining balanced testosterone levels through a healthy lifestyle and addressing any underlying medical conditions can greatly increase the chances of successful conception.

Follicle-Stimulating Hormone (FSH)

Follicle-Stimulating Hormone (FSH) plays a crucial role in male fertility and has a significant impact on the chances of conception. FSH is a hormone produced by the pituitary gland in the brain and is responsible for stimulating the production of sperm in the testicles.

FSH acts on the Sertoli cells in the testicles, which are essential for the development and maturation of sperm. It promotes the growth and division of the germ cells, which eventually develop into mature sperm. Without adequate levels of FSH, the production of sperm may be impaired, leading to reduced fertility.

Low levels of FSH can indicate a problem with the pituitary gland or hormonal imbalance, which can affect male fertility. On the other hand, high levels of FSH may indicate testicular dysfunction or damage, which can also hinder conception.

It is important to maintain a proper balance of FSH for optimal male fertility. Abnormal levels of FSH can affect the quality and quantity of sperm, making it more difficult to achieve pregnancy. Therefore, it is essential to monitor FSH levels and address any abnormalities to improve the chances of conception.

In some cases, fertility treatments may be recommended to regulate FSH levels and enhance male fertility. These treatments may include hormone therapy or assisted reproductive techniques such as in vitro fertilization (IVF).

In conclusion, Follicle-Stimulating Hormone (FSH) plays a vital role in male fertility and has a significant impact on the chances of conception. Maintaining proper FSH levels is crucial for the production and maturation of sperm, which are essential for successful fertilization. Monitoring FSH levels and addressing any abnormalities can help improve male fertility and increase the chances of conception.

Luteinizing Hormone (LH)

The luteinizing hormone (LH) plays a crucial role in male fertility and has a significant influence on successful conception. LH is produced by the pituitary gland and is responsible for stimulating the production of testosterone in the testes. Testosterone is essential for the development and maturation of sperm, as well as for maintaining overall reproductive health in men.

LH levels in the body fluctuate throughout the day, with the highest levels typically occurring in the morning. This hormone is released in response to signals from the hypothalamus, which senses the need for increased testosterone production. When LH levels rise, they trigger the release of testosterone from the testes, promoting the growth and development of sperm.

In addition to its role in testosterone production, LH also plays a crucial role in the process of ovulation in women. During the female menstrual cycle, LH levels surge, causing the release of a mature egg from the ovary. This egg must then be fertilized by sperm for conception to occur.

For successful conception to take place, it is important for LH levels to be within the normal range. Low levels of LH can indicate hormonal imbalances or issues with the pituitary gland, which may affect the production of testosterone and the maturation of sperm. On the other hand, high levels of LH may indicate conditions such as polycystic ovary syndrome (PCOS) in women or testicular dysfunction in men.

Monitoring LH levels can be helpful in assessing male fertility and identifying any underlying issues that may be affecting conception. This can be done through blood tests that measure the levels of various hormones, including LH. If LH levels are found to be abnormal, further evaluation and treatment may be necessary to improve fertility and increase the chances of successful conception.

In conclusion, LH plays a vital role in male fertility and has a significant influence on successful conception. It stimulates the production of testosterone, which is essential for the development and maturation of sperm. Monitoring LH levels can provide valuable insights into male fertility and help identify any hormonal imbalances or issues that may be hindering conception. By understanding the importance of LH and its impact on fertility, individuals and couples can take proactive steps to optimize their reproductive health and increase their chances of achieving pregnancy.

Sexual Health

Sexual health plays a crucial role in male fertility and the process of conception. It is essential for couples trying to conceive to have a healthy and satisfying sexual relationship. A strong connection between sexual health and male fertility exists, as both factors contribute to successful conception.

One important aspect of sexual health is erectile function. Erectile dysfunction, or the inability to achieve or maintain an erection, can have a significant impact on male fertility. It can hinder the ability to engage in sexual intercourse, making conception more challenging. It is essential for men experiencing erectile dysfunction to seek medical advice and explore potential treatments to improve their sexual health and increase their chances of conception.

Another factor to consider is the presence of sexually transmitted infections (STIs). STIs can have detrimental effects on male fertility and the ability to conceive. Infections such as chlamydia or gonorrhea can lead to inflammation and scarring of the reproductive organs, which can interfere with sperm production and motility. It is crucial for individuals to practice safe sex and get tested regularly to prevent the transmission of STIs and protect their sexual health.

Additionally, sexual frequency is an important aspect of male fertility. Regular sexual activity increases the chances of successful conception. Couples are advised to have intercourse every two to three days throughout the menstrual cycle to ensure that sperm is present during ovulation. Maintaining a healthy and active sex life is beneficial for both sexual health and the journey towards parenthood.

In conclusion, sexual health is closely linked to male fertility and the process of conception. Maintaining a healthy sexual relationship, addressing any issues related to erectile function, practicing safe sex, and ensuring regular sexual activity are all essential for couples trying to conceive. By prioritizing sexual health, individuals can increase their chances of successful conception and embark on the journey of parenthood.

Erectile Dysfunction

Erectile dysfunction (ED) is a common condition that affects many men and can have a significant impact on male fertility and the ability to conceive. ED refers to the inability to achieve or maintain an erection sufficient for sexual intercourse. This condition can arise from various factors, including physical, psychological, or a combination of both.

When it comes to male fertility, erectile dysfunction can pose challenges in the process of conception. The inability to achieve and sustain an erection can make sexual intercourse difficult or even impossible, thus hindering the chances of successful fertilization.

ED can have both physical and psychological effects on male fertility. Physically, the inability to achieve an erection can prevent sperm from being deposited in the vagina during intercourse, reducing the chances of sperm reaching and fertilizing an egg. Additionally, ED may also affect the quality of the sperm, leading to reduced fertility. Psychological factors such as stress, anxiety, and depression associated with ED can further impact fertility by affecting sexual desire and performance.

It is important for individuals experiencing erectile dysfunction to seek medical advice and treatment options. There are various treatment approaches available, including medication, lifestyle changes, and therapy, depending on the underlying cause of ED. By addressing and managing erectile dysfunction, individuals can improve their chances of conception and enhance their overall fertility.

Sexually Transmitted Infections (STIs)

Sexually Transmitted Infections (STIs) can have a significant impact on male fertility and the chances of conception. These infections are typically transmitted through sexual contact and can affect the reproductive system in various ways. It is important to understand the relationship between STIs and male fertility in order to take appropriate precautions and seek necessary treatment.

STIs such as chlamydia, gonorrhea, and syphilis can lead to inflammation and damage in the reproductive organs, including the testicles, epididymis, and prostate. This inflammation can interfere with the production and quality of sperm, reducing the chances of successful fertilization. In some cases, STIs can also cause scarring and blockages in the reproductive tract, further hindering the movement of sperm.

Additionally, certain STIs can cause hormonal imbalances in the body, affecting the production of testosterone and other hormones that are essential for male fertility. These hormonal disruptions can impact sperm production and function, making it more difficult to achieve conception.

It is important to note that not all STIs have the same impact on male fertility. The severity of the infection, the duration of the infection, and the promptness of treatment can all influence the potential consequences for fertility. Therefore, it is crucial to practice safe sex and undergo regular testing for STIs to prevent and address any potential issues.

In cases where an STI is detected, prompt treatment is essential to minimize the impact on fertility. Antibiotics are commonly prescribed to treat bacterial STIs, while antiviral medications may be used for certain viral infections. It is important to follow the prescribed treatment plan and complete the full course of medication to ensure complete eradication of the infection.

Overall, the relationship between STIs and male fertility is a complex one. Taking preventive measures, practicing safe sex, and seeking prompt treatment for any detected infections are crucial steps in maintaining reproductive health and maximizing the chances of successful conception.

Sexual Frequency

The role of sexual frequency in male fertility is an important factor to consider when trying to conceive. Regular sexual activity can significantly increase the chances of conception by ensuring that sperm is present in the reproductive system when the egg is released. When a couple is trying to conceive, it is recommended to have sexual intercourse every 2-3 days throughout the menstrual cycle. This ensures that the sperm count remains high and that there is a constant supply of sperm available for fertilization. Additionally, frequent sexual activity can also improve the quality of sperm. Regular ejaculation helps to flush out older sperm and replace them with fresh, healthy sperm. This can increase the chances of conception by ensuring that the sperm being released is of the highest quality. It is important to note that excessive sexual activity or the opposite, infrequent sexual activity, can have a negative impact on male fertility. Overly frequent ejaculation can deplete the sperm count, while infrequent ejaculation can lead to a decrease in sperm motility. In conclusion, maintaining a regular sexual frequency is essential for optimizing male fertility and increasing the chances of successful conception. By having regular sexual intercourse throughout the menstrual cycle, couples can maximize their chances of achieving pregnancy.

Lifestyle Factors

Lifestyle factors play a crucial role in male fertility and can significantly impact the process of conception. The choices we make in our daily lives, such as our habits, behaviors, and overall lifestyle, can have both positive and negative effects on male reproductive health.

One of the major lifestyle factors that can affect male fertility is smoking. Smoking has been found to have detrimental effects on sperm health, including decreased sperm count, motility, and morphology. The toxins present in cigarettes can damage the DNA in sperm cells, impairing their ability to fertilize an egg. Therefore, quitting smoking is essential for improving male fertility and increasing the chances of successful conception.

Another lifestyle factor that can impact male fertility is alcohol consumption. Excessive alcohol intake has been associated with decreased testosterone levels, impaired sperm production, and poor sperm quality. It is advisable for men trying to conceive to limit their alcohol consumption or avoid it altogether to optimize their fertility.

Diet and nutrition also play a significant role in male fertility. A healthy diet rich in essential nutrients, vitamins, and minerals can support optimal sperm production and function. Including foods high in antioxidants, such as fruits, vegetables, and nuts, can help protect sperm from oxidative damage and improve fertility. On the other hand, a poor diet lacking in essential nutrients can negatively affect sperm health and decrease the chances of conception.

Exercise and weight management are also important factors to consider for male fertility. Regular exercise has been shown to improve sperm quality and increase testosterone levels. However, excessive exercise or intense physical activity can have the opposite effect and negatively impact fertility. Maintaining a healthy weight is also crucial, as both obesity and being underweight can disrupt hormonal balance and impair sperm production.

By understanding the impact of lifestyle factors on male fertility, individuals and couples can make informed choices to optimize their chances of conception. Making positive changes in lifestyle habits, such as quitting smoking, moderating alcohol consumption, adopting a healthy diet, engaging in regular exercise, and maintaining a healthy weight, can significantly improve male fertility and increase the likelihood of successful conception.

Smoking

Smoking has been found to have detrimental effects on male fertility and can potentially hinder successful conception. The harmful chemicals present in cigarettes, such as nicotine and carbon monoxide, can negatively impact sperm production, sperm health, and hormonal balance.

Research has shown that smoking can lead to a decrease in sperm count, as well as a decrease in sperm motility and morphology. This means that smokers may have a lower number of sperm and a higher percentage of abnormal sperm, which can reduce the chances of successful fertilization and pregnancy.

In addition to affecting sperm quality, smoking can also disrupt hormonal balance in the body. It has been found to decrease testosterone levels, which can further impact male fertility. Testosterone is essential for the production of healthy sperm and plays a crucial role in the overall reproductive function.

Furthermore, smoking has been linked to erectile dysfunction, a condition that can make it difficult for men to achieve and maintain an erection. This can significantly affect the ability to conceive, as sexual intercourse is necessary for fertilization to occur.

It is important to note that the negative effects of smoking on male fertility are not limited to active smokers. Secondhand smoke exposure has also been associated with decreased sperm quality and fertility issues. Therefore, it is crucial for both men and their partners to avoid smoking and exposure to smoke to optimize their chances of successful conception.

Alcohol Consumption

Examining the influence of alcohol consumption on male fertility and its impact on the ability to conceive.

Alcohol consumption has long been a topic of debate when it comes to male fertility and conception. While enjoying a drink or two may seem harmless, excessive and chronic alcohol consumption can have detrimental effects on male reproductive health.

One of the main ways in which alcohol affects male fertility is by disrupting hormone production. Alcohol interferes with the normal functioning of the hypothalamus, pituitary gland, and testes, which are responsible for regulating hormone levels in the body. This disruption can lead to decreased testosterone production, impaired sperm development, and reduced sperm count.

Furthermore, alcohol has been shown to negatively impact sperm quality and motility. Studies have found that excessive alcohol consumption can cause abnormalities in sperm shape and structure, making it more difficult for them to reach and fertilize an egg. Additionally, alcohol can impair sperm motility, affecting their ability to swim effectively towards the egg for fertilization.

It is important to note that even moderate alcohol consumption can have an impact on male fertility. Research suggests that even as little as five alcoholic drinks per week can decrease sperm quality and quantity. Therefore, it is advisable for men who are trying to conceive to limit their alcohol intake or abstain from alcohol altogether.

Moreover, alcohol consumption can also affect sexual performance and erectile function. Excessive alcohol consumption can lead to erectile dysfunction, making it more challenging for couples to achieve successful intercourse and increase the chances of conception.

In conclusion, alcohol consumption can have a significant influence on male fertility and the ability to conceive. It is important for men to be aware of the potential risks associated with excessive alcohol consumption and make conscious choices to prioritize their reproductive health. By adopting a healthier lifestyle and reducing alcohol intake, men can improve their chances of successful conception and ultimately fulfill their dreams of starting a family.

Diet and Nutrition

When it comes to male fertility and conception, diet and nutrition play a crucial role. A healthy diet and proper nutrition are essential for maintaining optimal reproductive health and increasing the chances of successful conception.

A well-balanced diet that includes a variety of nutrient-rich foods can provide the necessary vitamins, minerals, and antioxidants that support sperm production and function. Certain nutrients, such as zinc, folate, vitamin C, vitamin E, and selenium, have been found to have positive effects on male fertility.

Zinc, for example, is important for sperm production and motility. Good sources of zinc include oysters, beef, poultry, beans, and nuts. Folate, found in leafy greens, citrus fruits, and fortified grains, has been associated with improved sperm quality. Vitamin C, abundant in fruits and vegetables, helps protect sperm from oxidative damage. Vitamin E, found in nuts, seeds, and vegetable oils, is known for its antioxidant properties and potential benefits for sperm health. Selenium, present in Brazil nuts, seafood, and eggs, is also believed to support sperm function.

In addition to specific nutrients, a healthy diet should also include an adequate intake of protein, healthy fats, and carbohydrates. Lean sources of protein, such as fish, poultry, and legumes, provide essential amino acids that are important for sperm production. Healthy fats, such as those found in avocados, olive oil, and nuts, can help regulate hormone production and improve sperm quality. Complex carbohydrates, like whole grains and fruits, provide energy and essential nutrients.

It's important to note that maintaining a healthy weight is also crucial for male fertility. Obesity has been associated with decreased sperm quality and hormonal imbalances, while being underweight can also have negative effects on fertility. A balanced diet and regular exercise can help achieve and maintain a healthy weight, which in turn can improve fertility outcomes.

In conclusion, a healthy diet and proper nutrition are vital for male fertility and conception. By incorporating nutrient-rich foods, maintaining a healthy weight, and adopting a balanced lifestyle, men can optimize their reproductive health and increase their chances of successful conception.

Exercise and Weight

Exercise and weight play a crucial role in male fertility and the process of conception. Maintaining a healthy weight through regular exercise is essential for optimizing fertility outcomes.

Exercise helps to improve overall health and well-being, which in turn positively impacts reproductive health. It helps to regulate hormone levels, improve blood circulation, and reduce stress levels, all of which are vital for optimal sperm production and function. Regular physical activity also helps to maintain a healthy body weight, which is important for fertility.

Studies have shown that excessive weight gain or obesity can have a negative impact on male fertility. Excess body fat can lead to hormonal imbalances, such as increased estrogen levels and decreased testosterone levels, which can impair sperm production and quality. It can also increase the risk of conditions such as erectile dysfunction and lower sperm count.

On the other hand, being underweight or engaging in excessive exercise can also negatively affect male fertility. Intense and prolonged physical activity can lead to the production of excessive amounts of free radicals, which can damage sperm cells. It can also disrupt hormone production and affect sperm quality. Therefore, it is important to strike a balance and engage in moderate exercise routines that promote overall health without overexertion.

In addition to exercise, maintaining a healthy weight through proper nutrition is equally important for male fertility. A balanced diet rich in essential nutrients, vitamins, and minerals can support optimal sperm production and function. It is recommended to include foods that are high in antioxidants, such as fruits and vegetables, as they help to protect sperm cells from oxidative damage. Adequate hydration is also essential for maintaining sperm health.

In conclusion, exercise and weight management play a significant role in male fertility and the process of conception. Regular exercise helps to improve overall health, regulate hormone levels, and maintain a healthy body weight, all of which are crucial for optimal sperm production and function. It is important to strike a balance and engage in moderate exercise routines while maintaining a healthy weight through proper nutrition. By prioritizing exercise and weight management, individuals can enhance their chances of successful conception.

Age and Fertility

Age and Fertility

One of the key factors that can significantly impact male fertility is age. As men age, their fertility levels gradually decline, which can have implications for the chances of conception. Understanding the correlation between age and fertility is crucial for couples who are planning to start a family.

Declining Fertility with Age

Research has shown that male fertility tends to decline as age advances. This decline is primarily attributed to a decrease in sperm quality and quantity. As men get older, the production of sperm may be affected, leading to lower sperm count and reduced motility. These factors can make it more challenging for couples to conceive.

Furthermore, advancing age in men has been linked to an increased risk of genetic abnormalities in their sperm. These genetic abnormalities can potentially impact the health and development of the resulting offspring. Therefore, it is essential for couples to be aware of the potential risks associated with advancing paternal age.

Advancing Paternal Age

While women have long been associated with the concept of a biological clock, studies have increasingly highlighted the importance of paternal age as well. Advanced paternal age has been linked to various fertility challenges and potential complications during pregnancy.

One significant concern associated with advancing paternal age is an increased risk of genetic disorders in offspring. As men age, the quality of their sperm may be compromised, leading to a higher likelihood of genetic mutations and chromosomal abnormalities. These mutations can increase the risk of conditions such as autism, schizophrenia, and certain syndromes in children.

Additionally, advancing paternal age has been associated with an increased risk of pregnancy complications, such as preterm birth and gestational diabetes. These risks can impact both the health of the mother and the baby.

Conclusion

Age plays a crucial role in male fertility and the chances of conception. As men age, their fertility levels gradually decline, impacting sperm quality, quantity, and genetic integrity. Couples should be aware of the potential challenges associated with advancing paternal age and take proactive measures to optimize their fertility and increase their chances of successful conception.

By understanding the impact of age on male fertility, couples can make informed decisions and seek appropriate medical guidance if needed. It is important to remember that age is just one factor among many that contribute to fertility, and every individual's situation is unique. Open communication, regular health check-ups, and a healthy lifestyle can all contribute to maintaining optimal fertility levels, regardless of age.

Declining Fertility with Age

As men age, their fertility naturally declines, which can have an impact on their ability to conceive. This decline in fertility is due to various factors that occur as the body ages. Understanding the effects of age on male fertility is crucial for couples trying to conceive.

One of the main reasons for declining fertility with age is a decrease in sperm count. As men get older, the production of sperm decreases, leading to a lower number of viable sperm available for fertilization. This decrease in sperm count can significantly reduce the chances of successful conception.

In addition to a decrease in sperm count, advancing age can also affect sperm motility. Sperm motility refers to the ability of sperm to move effectively towards the egg for fertilization. As men age, the motility of their sperm may decrease, making it more difficult for sperm to reach and fertilize the egg.

Furthermore, the quality of sperm can also be affected by age. Sperm morphology, which refers to the size and shape of sperm, can be negatively impacted as men age. Abnormal sperm morphology can hinder successful conception as it may affect the sperm's ability to penetrate the egg.

It is important for couples to be aware of the decline in male fertility with age and to consider this factor when trying to conceive. Seeking medical advice and exploring fertility treatments or assisted reproductive technologies can help overcome the challenges associated with declining fertility.

Advancing Paternal Age

Advancing paternal age refers to the increasing age of men at the time of conception. While it is widely known that a woman's age can affect her fertility, the impact of paternal age on conception is often overlooked. However, research has shown that advancing paternal age can have potential risks and implications for successful conception.

One of the main concerns associated with advancing paternal age is the increased risk of genetic abnormalities in offspring. As men age, the quality of their sperm may decline, leading to an increased likelihood of genetic mutations or chromosomal abnormalities. This can result in a higher risk of conditions such as Down syndrome and autism in children born to older fathers.

Additionally, advancing paternal age has been linked to an increased risk of certain medical conditions in offspring. Studies have found associations between older fathers and a higher incidence of conditions such as schizophrenia, bipolar disorder, and certain types of cancer in their children. While the exact mechanisms behind these associations are still being studied, it is believed that age-related changes in sperm DNA may play a role.

Furthermore, advancing paternal age can also impact the overall health and well-being of the child. Older fathers may have a higher likelihood of experiencing age-related health conditions such as cardiovascular disease or diabetes, which can indirectly affect the health of their offspring. Additionally, older fathers may have reduced energy levels and may find it more challenging to keep up with the demands of parenting.

It is important to note that while advancing paternal age may pose certain risks, it does not mean that older men cannot father healthy children. Many men successfully conceive and have healthy babies well into their later years. However, it is advisable for couples considering parenthood at an older age to consult with a healthcare professional to understand the potential risks and make informed decisions.

Medical Conditions

Medical conditions can have a significant impact on male fertility and can affect the chances of successful conception. Certain health issues can interfere with the reproductive system and hinder the ability to father a child. It is important for men to be aware of these conditions and seek appropriate medical attention if necessary.

One medical condition that can affect male fertility is varicocele. Varicocele is a condition characterized by the enlargement of veins within the scrotum. This can lead to decreased sperm production and quality, making it more difficult to conceive. Treatment options for varicocele include surgery or embolization to repair the affected veins and improve fertility.

Another factor that can impact male fertility is genetic disorders. Certain genetic conditions can affect sperm production or function, making conception more challenging. Examples of genetic disorders that can affect male fertility include Klinefelter syndrome and cystic fibrosis. Genetic testing may be recommended for couples experiencing difficulties conceiving to identify any underlying genetic issues.

Hormonal disorders can also have an impact on male fertility. Conditions such as hypogonadism, where the testes do not produce enough testosterone, can affect sperm production and quality. Thyroid disorders and pituitary gland issues can also disrupt hormonal balance and impact fertility. Treatment options for hormonal disorders may include hormone replacement therapy to restore normal hormone levels.

It is important for men to be aware of these medical conditions and seek appropriate medical care if they suspect they may be affecting their fertility. Consulting with a healthcare professional specializing in reproductive medicine can help identify any underlying issues and develop a treatment plan to improve fertility and increase the chances of successful conception.

Varicocele

Varicocele is a condition characterized by the enlargement of veins within the scrotum, specifically the veins that drain the testicles. This condition affects approximately 15% of men and is often associated with male infertility. Understanding the effect of varicocele on male fertility is crucial in identifying potential obstacles to successful conception.

When varicocele occurs, the increased blood flow and pooling of blood in the affected veins can lead to elevated testicular temperature. This rise in temperature can have a detrimental effect on sperm production and function. The heat generated by varicocele can impair the development and maturation of sperm, resulting in decreased sperm count, motility, and morphology.

Furthermore, the increased pressure caused by varicocele can disrupt the blood supply to the testicles, leading to reduced oxygen and nutrient delivery. This compromised blood flow can further contribute to impaired sperm production and function. The combination of elevated testicular temperature and reduced blood flow can significantly hinder the chances of successful conception.

It is important for individuals with varicocele to seek medical attention and explore potential treatment options. Surgical intervention, such as varicocelectomy, can help alleviate the effects of varicocele on male fertility. By correcting the abnormal blood flow and reducing testicular temperature, surgical treatment can improve sperm production and enhance the chances of conception.

In conclusion, varicocele is a condition that can have a significant impact on male fertility and hinder successful conception. Understanding the effect of varicocele on sperm production and function is crucial in addressing potential obstacles to fertility. Seeking medical advice and considering appropriate treatment options can help improve the chances of conception for individuals with varicocele.

Genetic Disorders

Genetic disorders can have a significant impact on male fertility and the chances of conception. These disorders can be inherited and may affect various aspects of reproductive health. Understanding the relationship between genetic disorders and male fertility is crucial for couples trying to conceive.

Genetic disorders can affect sperm production, sperm health, and hormonal balance, all of which play a vital role in male fertility. Certain genetic conditions can lead to abnormal sperm production or function, resulting in a decreased ability to fertilize an egg. Additionally, genetic disorders can disrupt the hormonal balance necessary for optimal fertility.

Some genetic disorders can also affect the structure and function of the reproductive organs, making conception more challenging. For example, conditions like Klinefelter syndrome and cystic fibrosis can impact the development of the testes and the production of healthy sperm.

In some cases, genetic disorders can also increase the risk of infertility due to the presence of chromosomal abnormalities. These abnormalities can lead to a higher likelihood of miscarriage or the inability to conceive altogether.

It is essential for individuals with a family history of genetic disorders to consult with a healthcare professional or a genetic counselor before attempting to conceive. They can provide valuable insights into the potential risks and help couples make informed decisions about their reproductive options.

In conclusion, genetic disorders can have a significant impact on male fertility and the chances of conception. Understanding the relationship between genetic disorders and male fertility is crucial for couples trying to conceive. Seeking professional guidance can help individuals navigate the complexities of genetic disorders and make informed decisions about their reproductive health.

Hormonal Disorders

Hormonal disorders can have a significant impact on male fertility and can greatly affect the ability to conceive. Hormones play a crucial role in the reproductive system, regulating sperm production and function. When there is an imbalance or disruption in hormone levels, it can lead to various fertility issues.

One common hormonal disorder that can affect male fertility is hypogonadism, which is characterized by low testosterone levels. Testosterone is essential for sperm production and the overall health of the reproductive system. When testosterone levels are low, it can lead to a decrease in sperm count, motility, and morphology, making it more difficult to achieve successful conception.

Another hormonal disorder that can impact male fertility is hyperprolactinemia, which is characterized by high levels of prolactin in the blood. Prolactin is a hormone that is primarily associated with lactation in women, but it also plays a role in male fertility. Elevated levels of prolactin can interfere with the production of testosterone and suppress sperm production, leading to infertility.

In addition to these hormonal disorders, conditions such as thyroid dysfunction and adrenal disorders can also affect male fertility. The thyroid gland produces hormones that regulate metabolism and energy levels, and any disruption in thyroid function can impact sperm production and quality. Adrenal disorders, such as Cushing's syndrome, can also disrupt hormone balance and affect fertility.

It is important for men experiencing hormonal disorders to seek medical attention and undergo hormone therapy if necessary. Hormone replacement therapy can help restore hormone levels to normal and improve fertility outcomes. However, it is crucial to consult with a healthcare professional specializing in reproductive medicine to determine the most appropriate treatment plan.

In conclusion, hormonal disorders can have a significant influence on male fertility and the ability to conceive. Imbalances or disruptions in hormone levels can lead to various fertility issues, including decreased sperm production and function. Seeking medical intervention and hormone therapy can help address these hormonal disorders and improve fertility outcomes.

Environmental Factors

Environmental Factors

Environmental factors play a crucial role in male fertility and can significantly impact the process of conception. Various external elements in our surroundings can affect sperm health and fertility, potentially hindering successful fertilization and pregnancy. Understanding these environmental factors is essential for couples trying to conceive and for individuals seeking to optimize their reproductive health.

Exposure to Chemicals:

Chemical exposure is one of the key environmental factors that can negatively affect male fertility. Many chemicals found in everyday products, such as pesticides, industrial pollutants, and certain household cleaners, have been linked to reduced sperm quality and quantity. These chemicals can disrupt hormonal balance, impair sperm production, and decrease sperm motility, all of which are vital for successful conception. It is crucial to minimize exposure to harmful chemicals by using natural and organic products whenever possible and adopting a cautious approach towards environmental toxins.

Radiation Exposure:

Radiation exposure is another environmental factor that can have a detrimental impact on male fertility. Prolonged exposure to ionizing radiation, such as that from X-rays, nuclear radiation, or occupational hazards, can damage sperm DNA and impair sperm function. This damage can lead to reduced sperm quality and motility, making it more challenging to achieve conception. It is essential for individuals working in occupations with potential radiation exposure to take necessary precautions and follow safety guidelines to minimize the risk to their reproductive health.

Overall Impact:

While it is challenging to completely avoid all environmental factors that may affect male fertility, being aware of their potential impact is crucial. Minimizing exposure to harmful chemicals, adopting a healthy and environmentally conscious lifestyle, and seeking medical advice when necessary can all contribute to optimizing male fertility and increasing the chances of successful conception. By understanding the role of environmental factors in male fertility, individuals and couples can take proactive steps to protect and enhance their reproductive health.

Exposure to Chemicals

Exposure to chemicals can have a significant impact on male fertility and the chances of successful conception. Chemicals found in various everyday products and environments can disrupt the delicate balance of hormones and affect sperm production, motility, and morphology. These chemicals, known as endocrine disruptors, can mimic or interfere with the body's natural hormones, leading to reproductive issues.

One common chemical that has been linked to male fertility problems is bisphenol A (BPA), which is found in plastic containers, food packaging, and thermal paper receipts. Studies have shown that BPA exposure can reduce sperm quality and motility, making it more difficult for sperm to reach and fertilize an egg.

In addition to BPA, pesticides and herbicides used in agriculture have also been associated with male fertility issues. These chemicals can accumulate in the body over time and disrupt hormonal balance, leading to decreased sperm count and abnormal sperm morphology.

Furthermore, certain industrial chemicals, such as phthalates and polychlorinated biphenyls (PCBs), have been found to have detrimental effects on male fertility. Phthalates, commonly found in plastics, can interfere with testosterone production and impair sperm quality. PCBs, which were once widely used in electrical equipment and other industrial applications, have been linked to reduced sperm count and motility.

It is important to note that the effects of chemical exposure on male fertility can vary depending on the duration and level of exposure. However, it is advisable to minimize exposure to chemicals as much as possible, especially for individuals who are trying to conceive. This can be done by opting for BPA-free products, choosing organic foods, and reducing exposure to pesticides and other harmful chemicals in the environment.

In conclusion, exposure to chemicals can have a detrimental effect on male fertility and the chances of successful conception. It is crucial to be aware of the potential risks associated with chemical exposure and take necessary precautions to minimize exposure. By doing so, couples can increase their chances of achieving a healthy pregnancy and welcoming a new life into the world.

Radiation Exposure

Radiation exposure is a significant factor that can affect male fertility and have an impact on the chances of conception. Exposure to high levels of radiation, whether from medical procedures or occupational hazards, can have detrimental effects on sperm production and quality.

When the body is exposed to radiation, it can damage the DNA within the sperm cells, leading to abnormalities and reduced fertility. Radiation can also affect the functioning of the testes, which are responsible for producing sperm. This disruption in sperm production can result in a lower sperm count and decreased motility, making it more difficult for fertilization to occur.

It is important to note that the effects of radiation exposure on male fertility can vary depending on the dose and duration of exposure. High levels of radiation, such as those experienced during cancer treatments like radiation therapy, can have a more significant impact on fertility compared to lower levels of exposure.

In addition to medical procedures, occupational hazards such as working in environments with high levels of radiation, such as nuclear power plants or certain industrial settings, can also pose a risk to male fertility. It is crucial for individuals working in these fields to take appropriate precautions to minimize their exposure and protect their reproductive health.

To mitigate the potential risks associated with radiation exposure, it is advisable to consult with a healthcare professional or fertility specialist. They can provide guidance on the best course of action, such as avoiding unnecessary radiation exposure or exploring alternative fertility options if conception becomes challenging.

In conclusion, radiation exposure can have a significant impact on male fertility and the chances of conception. It is essential to be aware of the potential risks and take appropriate measures to protect reproductive health, especially for individuals who are regularly exposed to high levels of radiation through medical procedures or occupational hazards.

Frequently Asked Questions

- **What is the role of male fertility in conception?**

The role of male fertility in conception is crucial. Without healthy sperm and proper hormonal balance, successful fertilization and pregnancy may be challenging.

- ## How does sperm production affect male fertility?

Sperm production is essential for male fertility. If there is a problem with sperm production, such as low sperm count or abnormal morphology, it can significantly impact the chances of conception.

- ## What factors contribute to healthy sperm?

Several factors contribute to healthy sperm, including proper nutrition, avoiding harmful substances like smoking and excessive alcohol consumption, and maintaining a healthy lifestyle.

- ## Why is sperm count important for male fertility?

Sperm count is important because it determines the number of sperm available for fertilization. A low sperm count can reduce the chances of successful conception.

- ## What is the role of sperm motility in conception?

Sperm motility refers to the ability of sperm to move effectively. Good sperm motility is crucial for sperm to reach and fertilize the egg, increasing the likelihood of conception.

- **How does sperm morphology affect male fertility?**

Sperm morphology refers to the size and shape of sperm. Abnormal sperm morphology can hinder successful fertilization and decrease the chances of conception.

- **What is the significance of hormonal balance in male fertility?**

Hormonal balance plays a vital role in male fertility. Proper levels of testosterone, follicle-stimulating hormone (FSH), and luteinizing hormone (LH) are necessary for healthy sperm production and function.

- **How does erectile dysfunction affect male fertility?**

Erectile dysfunction can impact male fertility by making sexual intercourse and ejaculation difficult. It can hinder the delivery of sperm to the egg, reducing the chances of conception.

- **What is the connection between sexually transmitted infections (STIs) and male fertility?**

  STIs can affect male fertility by causing inflammation or damage to the reproductive organs. They can also lead to sperm abnormalities or blockages, hindering successful conception.

- **Does sexual frequency affect male fertility?**

  Sexual frequency can influence male fertility. Regular sexual activity ensures a constant supply of fresh sperm, increasing the chances of successful fertilization.

- **How does smoking impact male fertility?**

  Smoking can negatively affect male fertility by reducing sperm count, motility, and morphology. It can also damage DNA in sperm, increasing the risk of infertility and miscarriages.

- **What is the influence of alcohol consumption on male fertility?**

  Excessive alcohol consumption can impair male fertility by reducing testosterone levels, affecting sperm production and function. It can also lead to erectile dysfunction and hormonal imbalances.

- **How does diet and nutrition affect male fertility?**

  A healthy diet and proper nutrition are essential for male fertility. Nutrient deficiencies or an unhealthy diet can negatively impact sperm quality and overall reproductive health.

- **What is the connection between exercise, weight, and male fertility?**

  Maintaining a healthy weight and engaging in regular exercise can positively influence male fertility. Obesity or excessive exercise can disrupt hormonal balance and impair sperm production.

- **Does age affect male fertility?**

  Yes, age can affect male fertility. As men age, sperm quality and quantity may decline, making conception more challenging. Advanced paternal age can also increase the risk of genetic disorders in offspring.

- **What is the impact of varicocele on male fertility?**

  Varicocele, an enlargement of the veins within the scrotum, can impair male fertility by increasing testicular temperature and affecting sperm production and quality.

- **How do genetic disorders influence male fertility?**

  Genetic disorders can impact male fertility by causing abnormalities in sperm production or function. They may also increase the risk of infertility or genetic issues in offspring.

- **What is the influence of exposure to chemicals on male fertility?**

  Exposure to certain chemicals, such as pesticides or industrial pollutants, can negatively affect male fertility by disrupting hormone levels, damaging sperm DNA, or impairing sperm production.

- **How does radiation exposure affect male fertility?**

  Radiation exposure, whether from medical treatments or occupational hazards, can harm sperm production and quality, leading to temporary or permanent infertility.

Have Questions / Comments?

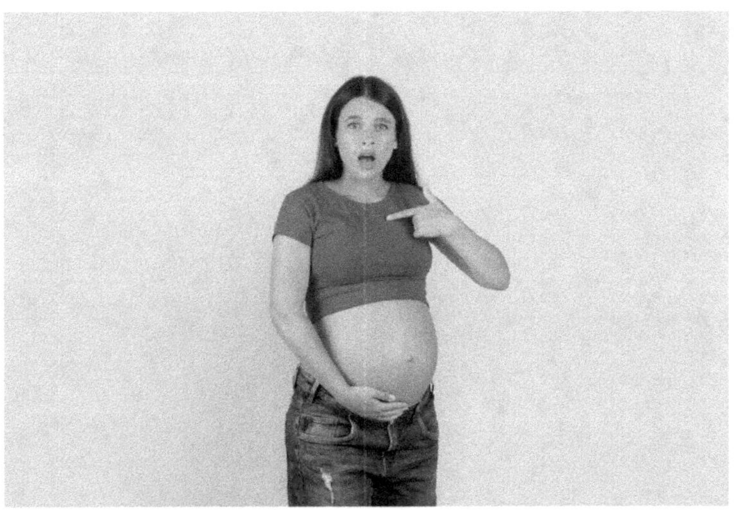

This book was designed to cover as much info as possible but I know I have probably missed something, or some new amazing discovery that has just come out.

If you notice something missing or have a question that I failed to answer, please get in touch and let me know. If I can, I will email you an answer and also update the book so others can also benefit from it.

Thanks For Being Awesome :)

Submit Your Questions / Comments At:

Get How To Be A Super Mom - 100% FREE

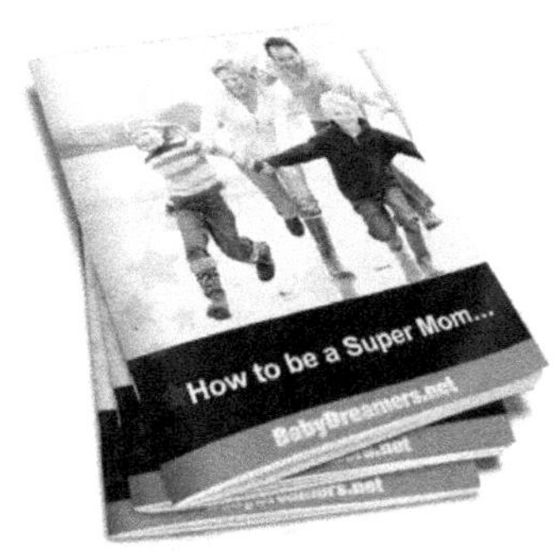

For being one of our amazing readers, we would love to offer you another book we have created, 100% free.

Being a mom is probably the most important job in the world – we've all heard that, and it's true. You're bringing up the next generation of wonderful, intelligent, loving, creative, responsible people.

We all want to be Super Mom and to be everything and do everything, but it this possible?

Being a Super Mom is possible, but you have to learn how to empower yourself to be the kind of Super Mom that you feel you need to be, keeping in mind that the title Super Mom doesn't mean the same thing to everyone.

Get How to be a Super Mom For Free at

BabyDreamers.net